MSWED

Gentle Pilates for the Golden Years

A Transformative Guide for Seniors

First edition

This book was professionally typeset on Reedsy.
Find out more at reedsy.com

Contents

Foreword

It is an honor and a privilege to offer these opening remarks to "Embracing Pilates in Senior Years" – a work of hope, renewal, and strength. Here before you is not simply an instructional volume; it is a lighthouse for all who navigate the latter passages of life's voyage, seeking to illuminate a path toward vitality, purpose, and grace.

As the writer of the foreword, it is my distinct pleasure to set the scene for what is undeniably an empowering journey. Together, from the first stretch to the final core-enhancing exercise, we will explore not just the how-tos but, more profoundly, the transformative powers of Gentle Pilates for those in the golden years.

The vision of this book is as straightforward as it is commendable: to shed light on the myriad benefits that Pilates offers seniors and to do so with a tone that speaks directly to the heart of this vibrant demographic. The golden years, often marked by reflection and transformation, are here re-imagined - they can, and should, be embraced with the kind of passion and vitality that Gentle Pilates promises.

The target audience—men and women stepping confidently into their 60s and beyond—will discover a guiding hand, a supportive voice, and a knowledgeable friend within these pages. Whether you're a seasoned Pilates practitioner or taking your very first steps into this world of mindful movement, this guide stands as your steadfast companion on a voyage to heightened well-being.

What follows in the ensuing chapters is a testimony to the resilience and adaptability of the human spirit. You will meet Martha, whose journey from skepticism to steadfast advocate for Pilates demonstrates this practice's universal appeal and applicability. Each subsequent chapter builds upon the last, intricately weaving together the technical know-how of Pilates with deeply personal narratives of triumph and steadfast dedication to health.

As the author of the foreword, I hope these preluding words will kindle within you a spark that will ignite a flame of curiosity, motivation, and resolve as you turn each page. And when the final words have been read, may that flame continue to burn brightly, guiding you through each day with the balance, strength, and harmony that Pilates can foster.

Journey onward, dear reader, and remember that within the realm of movement lies the promise of a life experienced fully and joyously. Welcome to your transformative journey through Gentle Pilates—let it be your guide to embracing the senior years with health, happiness, and an enduring zest for life.

Warm regards,

1

INTRODUCTION

Have you ever stood before a mirror, taking a moment just to marvel at the incredible machine that is your body, and wondered how to keep that machine running smoothly into your golden years? Imagine a key that can unlock a gentler, yet remarkably effective form of strength and vitality—a practice that can transform not only your physical state but also the way you move and feel in every facet of your life. This key is Pilates, and within these pages awaits a transformation journey uniquely suited to your unfolding story.

Abandoning the fluffy introductions and esoteric discussions that often clutter the path to practical knowledge, this book, "Gentle Pilates for the Golden Years: A Transformative Guide for Seniors," is structured with purpose at its heart. Each section is meticulously fashioned to deliver immediate value, guiding you toward an enhanced Pilates experience without a single wasted word.

Imagine a version of yourself with a stronger core, improved flexibility, and balance that gives you confidence with every step. Picture a life where every breath is deeper, each movement is smoother, and daily tasks are met with ease. By the time you complete this practice—not just in reading but in action—you'll not only have learned a series of exercises. You'll emerge with a newfound sense of control over your well-being, an embodiment of grace and strength, regardless of the year on your birth certificate.

As your hands turn these pages and your muscles embrace the discipline of Pilates, remember that this is more than a fitness regimen. It's a personal revolution. Pilates is the secret to a richer quality of life in your later years, a means by which to not just add years to your life, but life to your years. So, as you embark on this journey, do so knowing that you are equipped to make your golden years truly gleam with vitality and zest. Welcome to your transformative Pilates experience where every stretch, every breath, every movement is an investment in a vibrant, thriving future.

2

Understanding Pilates for Seniors and Its Main Goal

Personal Testimonial: Transformative Journey with Pilates

(Fictionalized for illustrative purposes)

Martha, a 68-year-old retiree, shares how Pilates helped her regain strength, improve balance, enhance posture, and foster new friendships.

> *"Joining a Pilates class was one of the best decisions I've made since retiring. After my 65th birthday, I could feel my body wasn't as strong as it used to be. I was slowly getting up from a chair and feared falling due to my poor balance. A friend suggested Pilates, and though I was skeptical at first, I soon proved wrong.*

> *Initially, I found it challenging, but the instructor adapted the exercises to my level, and I started noticing improvements in just a few weeks. My flexibility increased, and I felt more capable during my daily walks. Most incredibly, my family commented on how much straighter I was standing—no more slouching!>*

> *Pilates hasn't just enhanced my posture; it has transformed my life. I have better balance, am more muscular, and feel connected to*

my body in a way I haven't for years. But beyond the physical, it's the mental clarity and the friendships I've made in class that have been an unexpected yet invaluable gift. Now, I can't imagine my life without Pilates; it's a cornerstone of my health regime." - Martha, 68

—-

***Understanding Pilates for Seniors and Its Main Goal**:*
To appreciate the benefits for seniors, it's essential to understand Pilates and its main goal. Developed by Joseph Pilates in the early 20th century, Pilates transitioned from primarily a recovery tool to a versatile fitness method supporting seniors' well-being. Pilates, adaptable for seniors, aims to enhance the mind-body connection, supporting active aging through low-impact exercises (Latey, 2001).

The main goal of Pilates for seniors is to provide an accessible form of exercise that supports active aging. With low-impact, modifiable movements, Pilates meets the unique needs of this population, such as protecting joint health and minimizing the risk of chronic disease. Moreover, the group setting of many Pilates classes fosters a community atmosphere that can enhance emotional support and social interaction.

Benefits for Seniors:
Documented benefits include improved endurance, flexibility, balance, and posture—which are crucial for independence and fall prevention (Kloubec, 2010).

Mental Well-Being Enhancement:
Beyond these physical benefits, Pilates also contributes to

mental well-being. The mindful aspect of Pilates can yield stress relief and cognitive clarity (Donoyama & Ohkoshi, 2012).

In conclusion, Pilates represents a comprehensive approach for seniors to maintain a high quality of life, and it empowers individuals like Martha to navigate their golden years with strength, balance, and joy.

Quick Tips:
- *Start with gentle exercises.*
- *Focus on form and breathing.*
- *Regular practice fosters better results*

3

Preparing for Pilates

It is paramount to begin any new exercise program, including Pilates, with a clear understanding of health and safety considerations. This is why the initial step in preparing for Pilates is to consult a healthcare professional. Immediate emphasis on this critical action is not only prudent but essential. A healthcare provider can thoroughly assess an individual's medical history, current health condition, and specific requirements. With this professional guidance, one can confirm whether Pilates exercises are a suitable and safe option.

Highlighting the importance of medical advice before beginning Pilates (Wells, Kolt, & Bialocerkowski, 2012) investigated various dimensions of Pilates exercise, including its definition and systematic application. By grounding the practice of Pilates within a framework of expert health advice, individuals can identify potential risks or necessary modifications to the standard Pilates routine, tailoring it to their unique circumstances.

Finding the Right Instructor and Equipment
Seek certified instructors and consider the necessary equipment for a tailored Pilates experience.

In addition to securing medical clearance, a foundational step in preparing for Pilates involves finding an experienced and competent Pilates instructor. Qualified instructors can introduce novices to the core principles of Pilates, emphasizing correct form and technique to foster a safe and effective workout. Searching for the right instructor might entail researching credentials, surveying client testimonials, and participating in trial classes.

Once cleared by a healthcare professional and when an expert instructor is in place, it is time to consider the physical tools of the trade. While a mat is a standard for Pilates exercises, additional apparatuses such as the reformer, Cadillac, and Wunda chair can further refine one's practice. The Pilates instructor can recommend the most beneficial equipment based on individual goals and requirements.

Creating an environment conducive to focus and practice is crucial to acquiring the right equipment. This involves designating a peaceful, comfortable space that encourages concentration and dedication to the Pilates method. Proper workout attire that provides comfort and facilitates movement and the appropriate footwear for stability round out the preparations.

Lastly, mental readiness is instrumental in approaching Pilates with the appropriate mindset. Setting attainable goals, maintaining motivation, and practicing patience are all facets of mental preparation. Such an approach fosters progress and contributes to a satisfying and enriching Pilates journey.

In conclusion, Chapter 2 underscores the need to prioritize safety by consulting healthcare professionals and reinforces the necessity of qualified instruction, supportive equipment, a nurturing environment, and a focused mindset as essential components in preparing for Pilates. For elderly beginners and others alike, these guidelines provide the structure for a journey into Pilates that is both secure and fulfilling.

FAQ:
  - **Q:** How often should I practice Pilates?
  A: Start with 1-2 times per week.

- **Q:** Do I need special equipment?
  A: A mat suffices, but additional props can be beneficial

4

Breathing and Basic Pilates Principles

Breathing is a foundational element in Pilates that connects the mind to the body, facilitating fluid and efficient movements. Proper breathing helps to engage the core, maintain focused concentration, and ensure a harmonious practice. In essence, it fuels the practice of Pilates, ensuring that each movement is performed with maximum efficacy and safety.

The basic principles of Pilates — alignment, core engagement, and body awareness — are integral to the practice. Mastery of these principles is essential to derive the full benefits of Pilates, which include improved posture, muscle tone, and mental well-being.

Alignment:
Alignment refers to the proper positioning of the body parts. Correct alignment is crucial as it ensures that exercises are performed safely and effectively, preventing injury and allowing

for more efficient movement patterns.

Core Engagement:

The core comprises your abdomen, lower back, hips, and pelvis muscles. In Pilates, engaging these muscles is fundamental, as they provide stability and support for the entire body. Proper engagement aids in supporting the spine and maintaining good posture.

Body Awareness:

Body awareness involves being mindful of the positioning and movement of the body in space. It allows for greater control over movements and helps to correct form during exercises. This leads to more precise and fluid motions essential in Pilates practice.

Breathing Techniques

Steps for proper Pilates breathing are outlined to help seniors maximize exercise benefits.

1. **Find a Comfortable Position:**

Begin by lying on your mat with your knees bent and feet flat on the floor, or sit comfortably. Ensure your spine is in a neutral position, with your pelvis and shoulders in alignment.

2. **Inhale through the Nose:**

Breathe in slowly through your Nose, allowing your rib cage to expand laterally into your back and sides. This type of breathing is called "lateral thoracic breathing," it is essential for maintaining core engagement while allowing the ribs to move.

3. **Engage the Core:**

As you inhale, focus on engaging your core muscles. Imagine pulling your belly button towards your spine gently. Do not hold your breath, but maintain engagement of the abdominal.

4. **Exhale through the Mouth:**

Slowly exhale through your Mouth as if you are blowing through a straw. As you exhale, deepen the engagement of your core muscles and feel the abdominal contraction. Ensure that your neck and shoulders remain relaxed, and avoid shrugging.

5. **Continue the Breathing Cycle:**

Repeat this cycle of inhaling through the Nose and exhaling through the Mouth several times. Please pay attention to the rhythm of your breath and try to keep it steady and controlled.

6. **Incorporate Movement:**

Once you are comfortable with the breathing technique, incorporate it into your Pilates exercises. Exhale during the effort phase of the exercise (usually when you move against gravity), and inhale during the release phase.

7. **Practice Consistently:**

Like any other Pilates principle, breathing techniques require practice. Make proper breathing an integral part of your Pilates sessions and aim for consistency to benefit your physical and mental state during workouts.

Integrating proper breathing with the principles of alignment, core engagement, and body awareness will enhance your Pilates practice, achieving a more effective workout and a greater sense of well-being.

Incorporating these Pilates breathing techniques into your practice can significantly enhance the effectiveness of your workouts. Here's a sidebar for quick reference to common queries about Pilates breathing:

—-

FAQ

***Q:** Can I practice Pilates breathing outside of class?*
***A:** Yes, and it's encouraged!*

Frequently Asked Questions about Pilates Breathing

Q: Why is breathing so important in Pilates?

A: Breathing is essential in Pilates as it helps to activate the core, improve oxygenation of the muscles, and maintain focused concentration. It enhances the connection between mind and body, facilitating fluid and more efficient movements.

Q: What is lateral thoracic breathing?

A: Lateral thoracic breathing is a technique used in Pilates where you breathe deeply into the sides and back of your rib cage, expanding it laterally. This method helps keep the core engaged while allowing the chest to expand and contract during breathing.

Q: How does proper breathing affect core engagement in Pilates?

A: Proper breathing techniques enhance core engagement by teaching to contract your abdominal muscles as you exhale. This contraction provides excellent stability and support for your spine and pelvis during Pilates exercises.

Q: Are there any risks if I don't breathe correctly during Pilates?
A: Incorrect breathing can lead to insufficient oxygenation of the muscles, increased tension in the neck and shoulders, and can undermine the effectiveness of your core engagement. Over time, it may also increase the risk of injury.

Q: Can I practice Pilates breathing outside of my regular workouts?
A: Yes, practicing Pilates breathing throughout the day can improve posture, reduce stress, and increase awareness of your body's alignment and movements.

Remember that regular practice and being mindful of your body's response will allow you to refine your breathing over time, making your Pilates practice more rewarding and effective.

5

Building Core Strength

Understanding and enhancing core strength, particularly for seniors. This chapter emphasizes the
significance of a strong core for maintaining balance,
ensuring stability, and performing daily tasks efficiently. It
outlines a series of Pilates-based exercises tailored to meet the
needs of older adults aiming to fortify their core muscles.

Introduction to the Concept of the Core and Its Importance in Everyday Movements

The core is often thought of as the powerhouse of the body. It
consists of muscles that stabilize and support the spine, pelvis,
and shoulder girdle, forming a solid base for movement. A
robust core provides the foundation for all activities, ranging
from simple tasks such as standing and sitting with good
posture to more complex movements like bending, twisting,
and even walking. For seniors who may experience a natural
decline in muscle strength and stability, the core's strength

becomes even more paramount, as it ensures a balanced and stable body, reducing the risk of falls and supporting overall mobility and functionality.

Detailed instructions, illustrations, and modifications for three core-strengthening exercises are provided, targeting senior needs and abilities.

Pilates is particularly beneficial for seniors due to its gentle approach, emphasizing mindful movement and proper breathing techniques. This chapter will focus on specific Pilates exercises that have been shown to enhance core strength in older individuals effectively:

Here are more detailed instructions for three Pilates core-strengthening exercises tailored to seniors. These descriptions will include setup, movement, key points to remember, and modifications as needed.

Pelvic Curl:

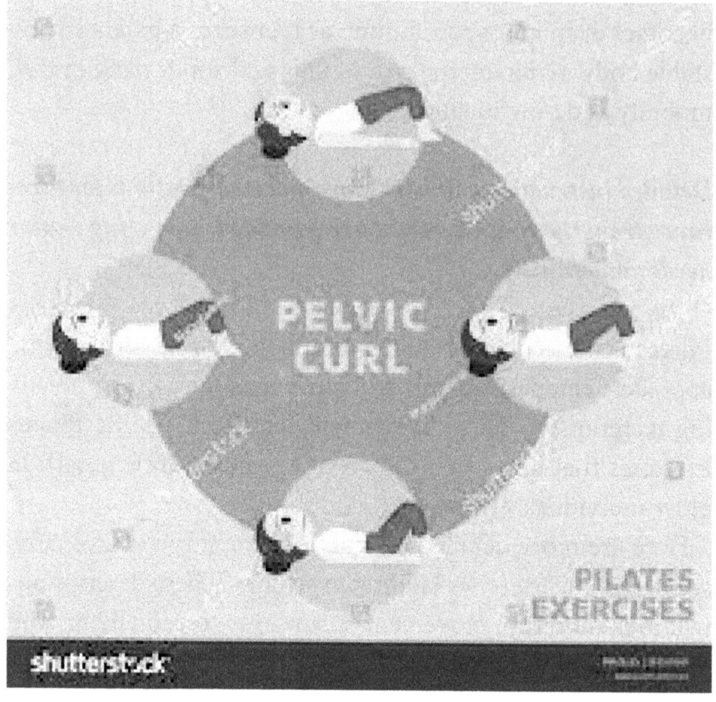

illustration: Pelvic Curl

SETUP

Lie on a mat with your knees bent, feet flat on the floor, and arms by your sides. Maintain a neutral spine with a natural curve in your lower back.

MOVEMENT

1. Start by inhaling to prepare. As you exhale, slowly tuck your pelvis and flatten your back against the mat, peeling your spine off the floor, beginning with the tailbone and progressing up the spine until you reach your shoulders.

2. Hold the position at the top for a breath, ensuring your

body forms a straight line from shoulders to knees.

3. Inhale at the top, and then as you exhale, gradually roll your spine back down onto the mat, one vertebra at a time, starting from your upper back and finishing with your tailbone to return to the starting position.

KEY POINTS

- Press your feet firmly onto the floor.
- Engage your abdominal muscles to lift your spine.
- Do not over-arch your back at the top of the movement; keep your hips aligned with your knees and shoulders.
- Move with control, articulating your spine.

MODIFICATION

Do not lift as high if you have difficulty keeping your hips elevated or experience back discomfort. Also, march your feet slightly wider apart to increase stability.

Chair-assisted Side Bends:

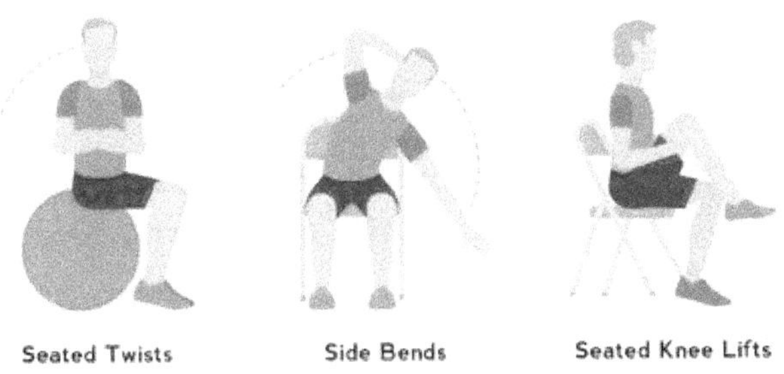

illustration: Chair-assisted Side Bends

SETUP

Sit on a chair with your feet flat on the floor, hip-width apart. Keep your back straight and maintain good posture throughout the exercise.

MOVEMENT

1. Raise one arm overhead; let the other hang by your side or rest on your hip.

2. Inhale to prepare, and as you exhale, bend your spine to the side, moving over the arm at your hip. Imagine you are between two panes of glass, keeping your bend strictly lateral without leaning forward or backward.

3. Inhale as you return to the starting upright position.

4. Repeat on the other side by switching your arms.

KEY POINTS

- Keep your shoulders relaxed and away from your ears.
- Only bend as far as comfortable; you should feel a stretch but no pain.
- Keep your hips square and seated firmly on the chair; avoid lifting them off the seat.

MODIFICATION

If you find raising your arm overhead too challenging, you can keep both hands on your hips and focus on the side bend with your torso.

Seated Twists:

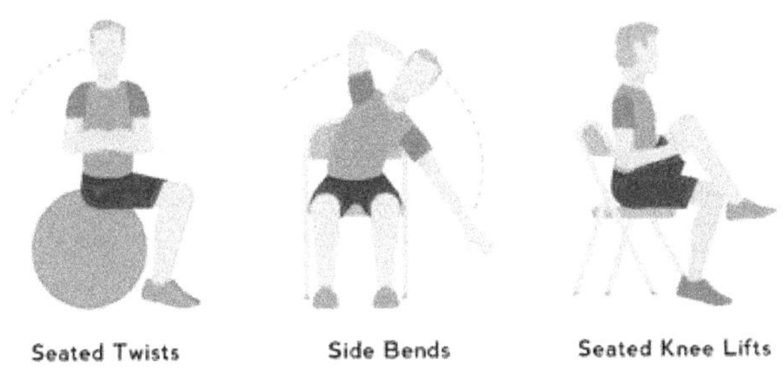

illustration: Seated twist

SETUP

Sit on a chair or ball with your feet flat on the floor and your hands behind your head or across your chest.

MOVEMENT

1. Inhale to prepare, sitting tall with your spine lengthened.

2. As you exhale, rotate your torso to one side, keeping your hips stationary and allowing the twist to come from your waist.

3. Hold the twist for a breath, then inhale as you gently return to the center.

4. Repeat on the opposite side.

KEY POINTS

- Keep your movements slow and controlled.

- Do not jerk or force the twist; it should be a gentle rotation.

- Engage your core muscles throughout the movement to support your spine.

MODIFICATIONS

Reduce the range of motion if you feel discomfort, or perform the exercise without the hands behind the head if it creates tension in the neck.

6

Improving Balance and Stability

T*he Importance for Seniors*
Balance enhances mobility, reduces fall risk, and improves an independent lifestyle.

As individuals age, maintaining good balance and stability becomes increasingly important. This is because balance and stability are critical factors in preventing falls, which are a leading cause of injury and loss of independence among seniors. Poor balance and stability can result from several aging factors, such as the deterioration of the vestibule system (inner ear balance mechanism), reduced muscle strength, limited joint mobility, and slower reflexes.

Pilates Role

Emphasizes core strength, mind-body connection, and adaptability—critical factors in balance improvement.

Pilates is a form of exercise that emphasizes controlled movements and core strength, making it particularly beneficial for improving balance and stability. Here's how:

1. **Core Strengthening:** Pilates focuses on strengthening the muscles of the core (the abdomen, lower back, hips, and pelvis). A strong core is essential for maintaining good posture and balance, providing a stable center of gravity.

2. **Mind-Body Connection:** Pilates requires concentration, coordination, and a deep connection between the mind and the body. This enhances proprioception, the body's ability to sense its position in space and adjust accordingly.

3. **Low-Impact Exercise:** Pilates is generally low-impact, making it a safe choice for seniors at risk of injury from more strenuous exercise.

4. **Flexibility and Joint Health:** Pilates movements help increase flexibility and range of motion, which is essential for keeping the joints healthy and improving overall stability.

5. **Balance Training:** Pilates includes exercises challenging the body's balance systems. These can range from simple exercises on the mat to more advanced movements using equipment like the Pilates reformer or wobble board.

6. **Adaptability:** Pilates exercises can be modified to suit different fitness levels and mobility issues, allowing seniors to start with more accessible variations and gradually progress as their balance and stability improve.

By participating in Pilates, seniors can improve their balance and stability, which will help reduce the risk of falls and injuries, increase confidence in performing daily activities, and promote a more active and independent lifestyle as they age.

Warning
- *Progress at your own pace.*
- *Use supports (like a chair) when necessary.*

7

Increasing Flexibility and Range of Motion

njury Prevention

Flexibility is vital for preventing injuries and maintaining everyday mobility.

Losing flexibility is expected as you age and can limit joint movement and make muscles stiff, making everyday tasks harder and increasing injury risk. Regular stretching exercises can keep muscles flexible and joints moving well to prevent falls and injuries.

Exercises for Seniors

Pilates suits seniors because it can be adjusted for different fitness levels and helps stretch muscles slowly, improving flexibility and relaxing muscles through controlled breathing.

The spine twist, cat stretch, and swan exercises are explained for enhancing flexibility in seniors.

Pilates Exercise Instructions

1. **Spine Twist**: Sit with legs out and arms to the side at shoulder height. Breathe in and elongate the spine, then twist the torso to one side while exhaling without moving the hips. Inhale to the center and repeat on the other side, doing five twists each way.

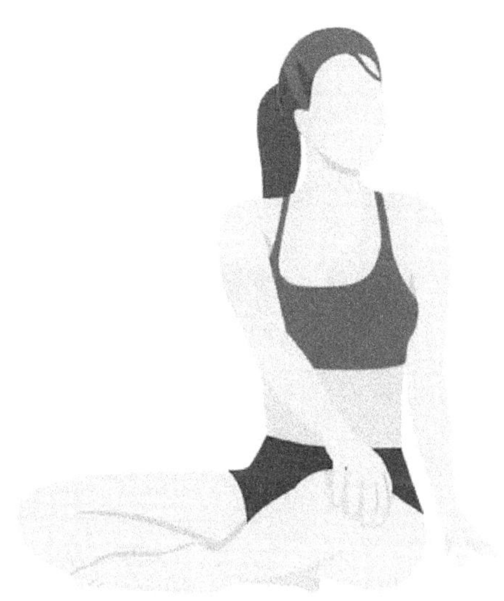

illustration: **Spine Twist**

2. **Cat Stretch**: On hands and knees, align your wrists

under your shoulders and knees under your hips. Inhale and let the belly drop, looking up. Exhale, pull the belly in and curve the back upwards. Do this for ten breath cycles.

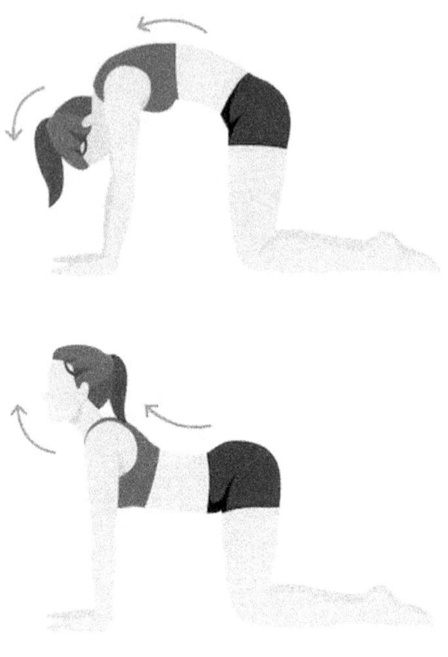

illustration: **Cat Stretch**

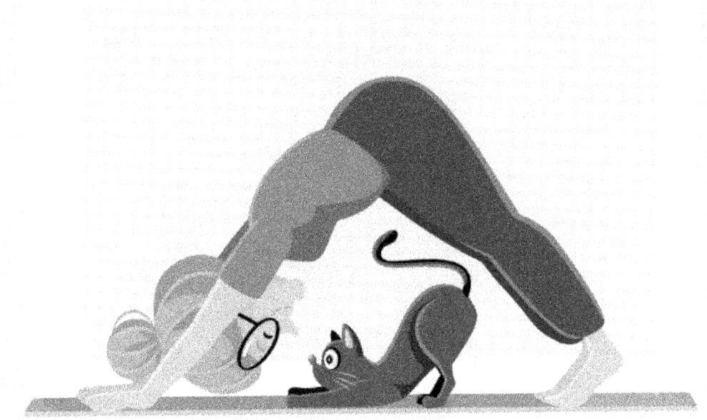

illustration: **Cat Stretch**

3. **Swan**: Lie on your stomach with hands under your shoulders and elbows close to the body. Use your abs to protect your back. Inhale and lift the head and chest, keeping the back bend slight. Exhale to lower back down. Do 5-8 times.

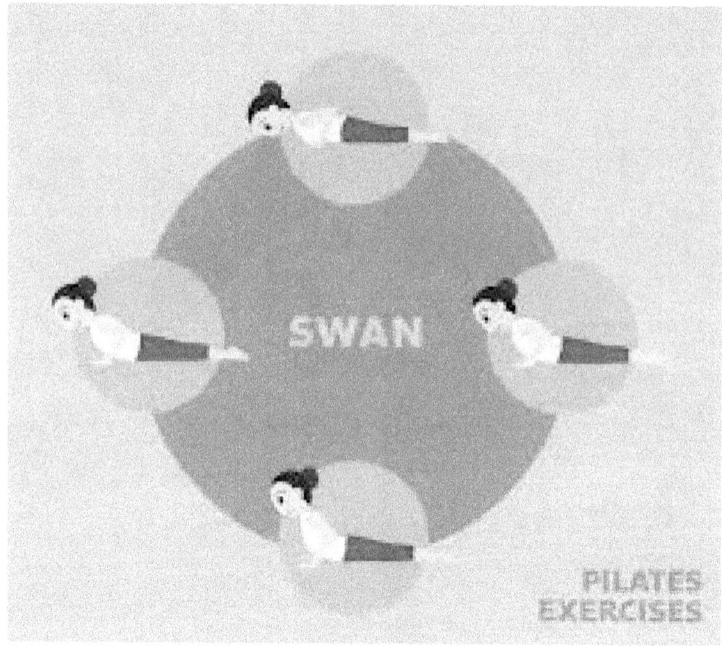

illustration: **Swan**

Seniors should talk to a doctor before starting exercises and consider finding a Pilates instructor with experience teaching older adults to ensure safety and proper technique.

Modification:
 - *All exercises can be modified for comfort and safety*

8

Enhancing Posture and Alignment

A. Addressing Postural Changes

Acknowledges the inevitability of postural changes with age and how Pilates can counteract these.

As individuals age, numerous factors contribute to changes in posture and alignment. Age-related changes in the muscles, bones, and joints can reduce flexibility, strength, and overall mobility. For instance, intervertebral discs may lose hydration and elasticity, leading to decreased spinal height and potential curvature. Osteoporotic changes can alter the structural integrity of bones, making fractures more likely.

Muscle weakness, particularly in the core and postural muscles, can lead to instability, increased risk of falls, and changes in gait. The weakening of the abdominal muscles, combined with a propensity for tighter chest muscles and forward head posture, can lead to a stooped posture, often called kyphosis.

B. Explanation of how Pilates can help improve posture and alignment for seniors

Pilates is a low-impact exercise that focuses on strengthening the core, including the abdomen, lower back, hips, and pelvis. By supporting these central muscles, Pilates helps seniors maintain better control over their posture. Pilates also emphasizes alignment, balance, and proper movement patterns, which can benefit aging individuals.

The practice of Pilates encourages the elongation of the spine and the strengthening of the muscles responsible for upright posture. It promotes awareness of body positioning, which is pivotal for correcting postural habits that may have developed over the years. Pilates exercises are also scalable, meaning they can be modified to accommodate varying fitness and mobility levels, making it an accessible form of exercise for most seniors.

C. *Pilates for Better Posture*

Three Pilates exercises with step-by-step instructions are shared to promote alignment and posture.

1. *Shoulder Bridge:*

- Lie flat on your back with your knees bent and feet flat on the floor, hip-width apart.
   - Place your arms by your sides with palms facing down.

- Inhale to prepare, exhale, and slowly roll your spine off the floor, lifting your hips towards the ceiling.

- Press down through your feet, engaging your glutes and hamstrings.

- At the top of the bridge, inhale and hold the position, ensuring your body forms a straight line from shoulders to knees.

- Exhale as you slowly roll your spine back onto the mat, one vertebra at a time.

- Repeat for 8-10 repetitions, focusing on smooth movement and stabilizing your pelvis.

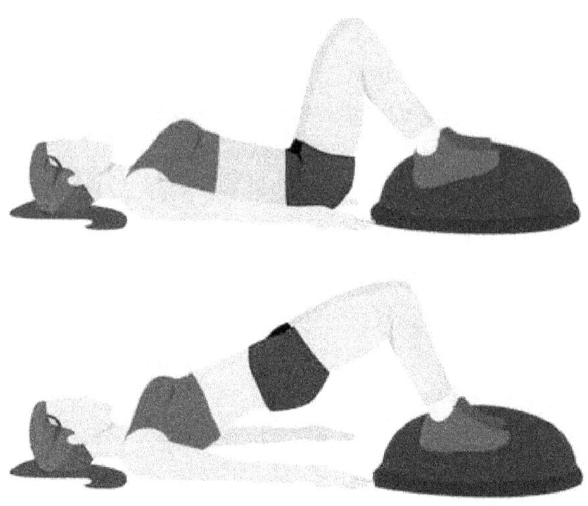

Illustration: **Shoulder Bridge**

2. Spine Stretch Forward:

- Sit up tall on a mat with your legs extended out in front of you, slightly wider than hip-width apart.

- Reach your arms out in front of you at shoulder height, palms facing down.

- Inhale to prepare, then exhale as you slowly curl your head and upper spine forward, reaching your fingertips towards your toes while keeping your abdominals scooped.

- Imagine peeling your spine off a wall, vertebra by vertebra, to encourage a more significant stretch.

- Inhale and stack your spine back up to the sitting position, from the lower back to the top of your head.

- Repeat the stretch 5-7 times, focusing on elongating the spine and creating space between the vertebrae.

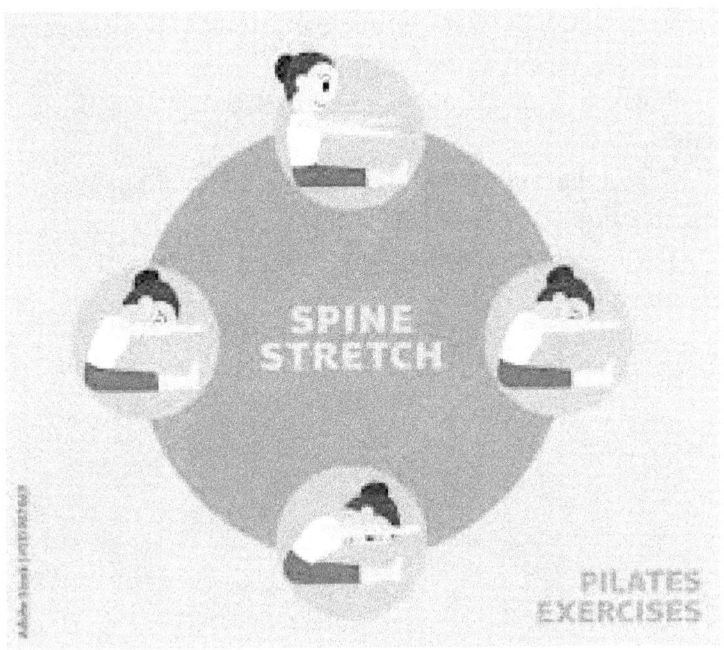

Illustration: **Spine Stretch Forward**

3. Pilate Saw:

- Sit with your legs spread wide and your arms stretched to the sides at shoulder height.

- Inhale, lengthening your spine, and as you exhale, rotate your torso to the right, reaching your left hand towards your right foot and your right hand in the opposite direction – in a 'sawing' motion.

- Keep your hips grounded and twist from the waist, turning your head to look at your backhand.

- Inhale as you unwind, coming back to center with a tall spine.

- Repeat the twist to the opposite side, and continue alternating sides for 8-10 repetitions on each side.

- Focus on the rotation of your spine and ensure that your movement is controlled and deliberate.

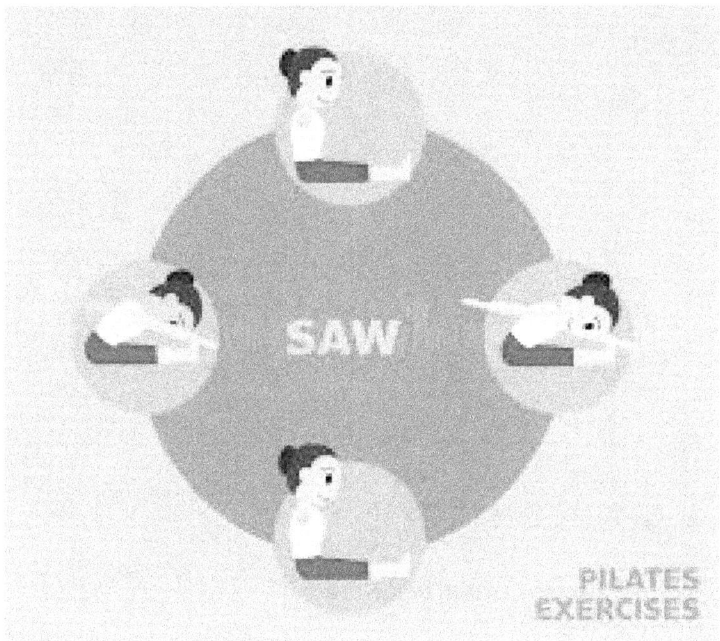

illustration: **Pilate Saw**

It is always essential for seniors to consult with a healthcare provider before starting any new exercise regimen, particularly if they have any existing health concerns or mobility limitations. Qualified Pilates instructors can also provide personalized guidance and modifications to ensure safety and effectiveness in improving posture and alignment.

Motivation:
   - Celebrate minor improvements.
   - Consistency leads to progress

9

Modifying Pilates Exercises for Individual Abilities

Listening to Your Body

This chapter Stresses the importance of modification and provides examples such as seated leg lifts and props for support.

Tips for adapting Pilates exercises for different abilities

Variations for seated exercises

Transferring exercises typically done lying down or standing to a seated position can lower the difficulty level and provide a safer option for those who struggle with balance or have limitations in standing for prolonged periods. For example, performing leg lifts while securely seated helps maintain core engagement and leg strength without the risk of falling.

Using props for support

Props can significantly enhance both the accessibility and the effectiveness of Pilates exercises. A Pilates ring can be squeezed between the thighs during a bridge to help activate the inner thigh muscles more intensively. At the same time, a foam roller can be used under the back during abdominal exercises to provide additional support and challenge core stability. Resistance bands can offer graduated resistance, so the tension can be adjusted to suit one's strength level. Additionally, supporting oneself with a chair or ballet barre during standing exercises can increase confidence and stability, allowing for better form and muscle engagement.

Structured Progression

Offers guidance for gradually increasing Pilates challenges, emphasizing safety and individual ability.

Increasing the challenges in a Pilates practice is critical to continued improvement and motivation. As referenced in *Clinical Interventions in Aging* structured and gradual increments in Pilates, such as longer holds, increased repetition, or incorporating more advanced positions, can have significant impacts on an individual's balance and functional capacity, particularly in older adults (Küçükçakır et al., 2013). Regular assessment by a qualified Pilates instructor can help tailor the progression to one's needs, ensuring each step is appropriately challenging without overwhelming or discouraging.

It is also essential to incorporate multidimensional progress, which includes not only intensity and complexity but also the refinement of the movements and the development of mind-body awareness. Monitoring one's comfort and fitness levels is crucial, and a professional can provide feedback on form, offer appropriate modifications, or introduce new exercises to suit evolving capabilities.

Examples of modifications for Pilates exercises

1. Seated Leg Lifts: Instead of performing leg lifts while lying down or standing, individuals can achieve them while securely seated. This modification helps maintain core engagement and leg strength without the risk of falling for those who struggle with balance or have limitations in standing for prolonged periods.

2. Bridge with Pilates Ring: To make the bridge exercise more accessible and activate the inner thigh muscles more intensively, individuals can squeeze a Pilates ring between their thighs while performing the bridge. This prop provides support and adds an extra challenge.

3. Abdominal Exercises with Foam Roller: Placing a foam roller under the back during abdominal exercises can provide additional support and challenge core stability. The foam roller acts as a prop, allowing individuals to maintain proper form and engage their core muscles effectively.

4. Adjustable Resistance Bands: Resistance bands are a versatile tool that can offer graduated resistance. Individuals can adjust the tension of the bands to suit their strength level. This modification allows for a personalized challenge and accommodates individual abilities.

5. Using a Chair or Ballet Barre for Support: Individuals who need assistance with balance and stability can use a chair or ballet barre for support during standing exercises. This provides added confidence and strength, allowing for better form and muscle engagement.

6. Structured Progression: Increasing the challenges in Pilates practice is essential for continued improvement and motivation. This can include longer holds, increased repetition, or incorporating more advanced positions gradually. Working with a qualified Pilates instructor who can assess individual needs and tailor the progression accordingly is essential.

7. Multidimensional Progress: Progression in Pilates should focus on intensity and complexity, refinement of movements, and development of mind-body awareness. Individuals should monitor their comfort and fitness levels and seek feedback from a professional to ensure proper form, appropriate modifications, and the introduction of new exercises that suit their evolving capabilities.

These modifications ensure that exercises are adapted to individual abilities, promoting safety, accessibility, and continued progress in Pilates practice.

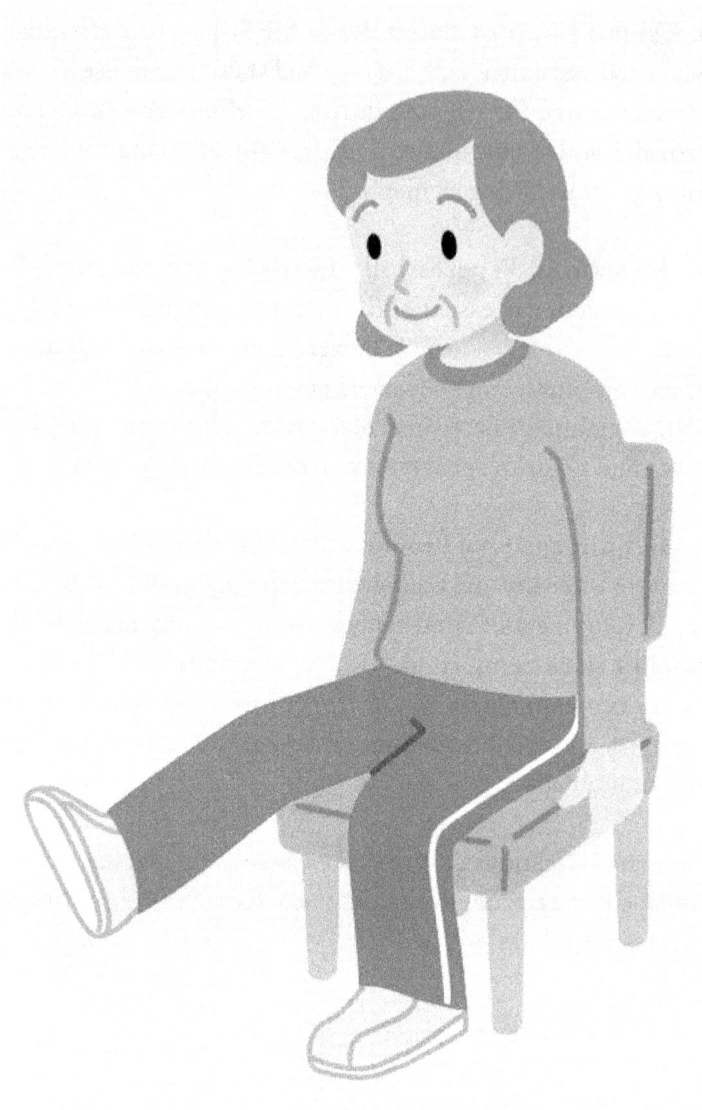

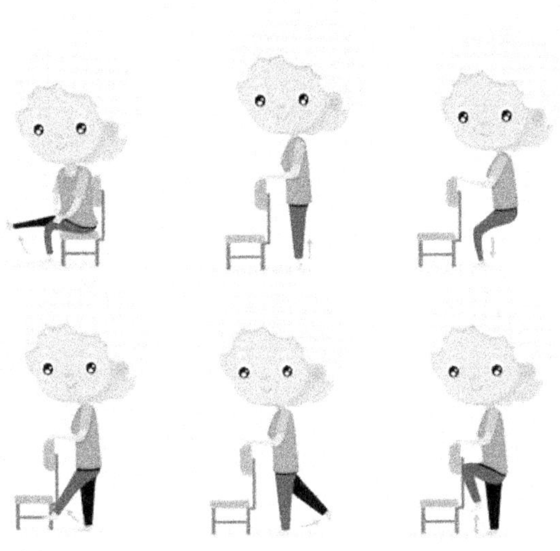

Tips
- *Props like chairs add stability.*
- *Recognize and respect your limits and progress slowly.*

10

Tailoring Pilates for the Elderly Beginner

The journey into Pilates as an elderly beginner can be rewarding and life-enhancing. With your golden years comes an opportunity to focus on health and well-being, and Pilates offers a gentle yet effective method to maintain physical strength, flexibility, and mental acuity. The key to reaping the full benefits lies in the consistent and regular practice of Pilates exercises, seamlessly integrating them into your daily life.

A. The Power of Consistency and Regularity

Integrating Pilates into your routine is crucial for enjoying its long-term benefits, which include improved posture, better balance, increased core strength, and enhanced mental well-being. Consistency helps build muscle memory, reinforcing the mind-body connection that Pilates is famed for, while regularity ensures that these benefits accumulate over time. As an elderly beginner, aim for frequent short sessions rather than sporadic longer ones, allowing your body to adapt to the new regimen without exhaustion.

B. Weaving Pilates into Your Daily Routines

Incorporating Pilates into your routine doesn't have to be daunting. Start by dedicating a specific time each day, whether in the quiet of the morning or the calm of the evening, to practice. Morning rituals may involve simple stretches and breathing exercises to awaken the body and promote circulation. Evening sessions could focus on winding down with exercises that relax the muscles and soothe the nervous system. Embedding Pilates exercises into everyday activities, like practicing balance while brushing your teeth or engaging your core during light housework, also ensures that your Pilates practice extends beyond designated workout times.

C. Staying Motivated and Complementary Activities

Staying motivated as an elderly beginner can be challenging. To maintain enthusiasm, set achievable goals, track progress, and reward milestones. Engage with a supportive community in person or online to share experiences and stay motivated through collective encouragement. To supplement your Pilates routine, consider physical activities that align with its principles, such as walking, swimming, or tai chi. These activities promote overall health without overstraining the body and complement the strength and flexibility developed through Pilates. Remember, every bit of movement counts, and keeping your body engaged will help you get the most out of your Pilates journey.

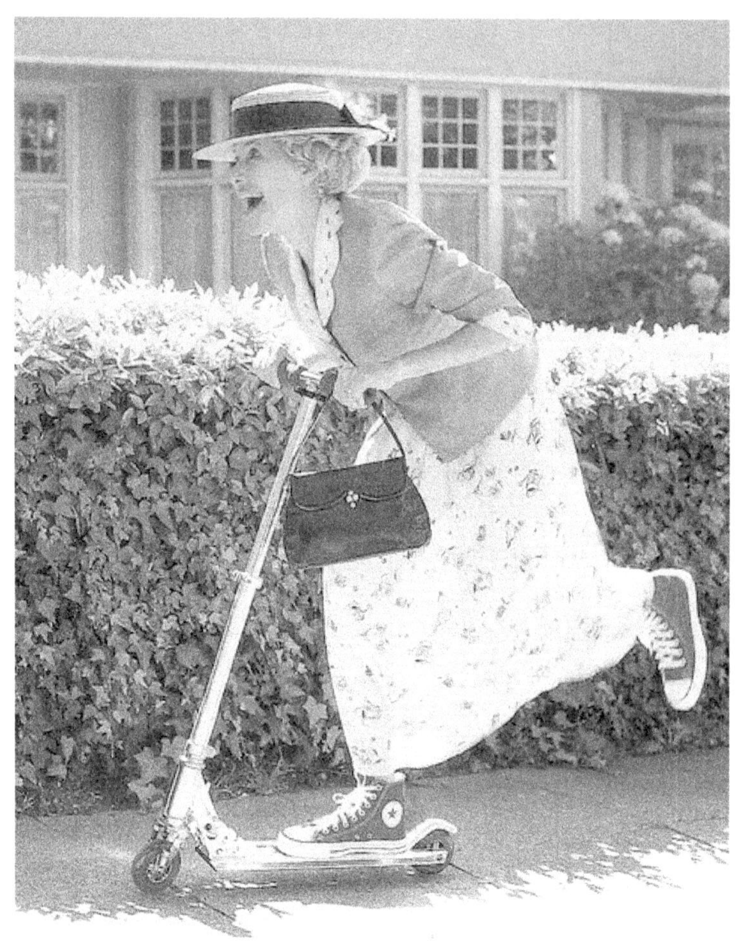

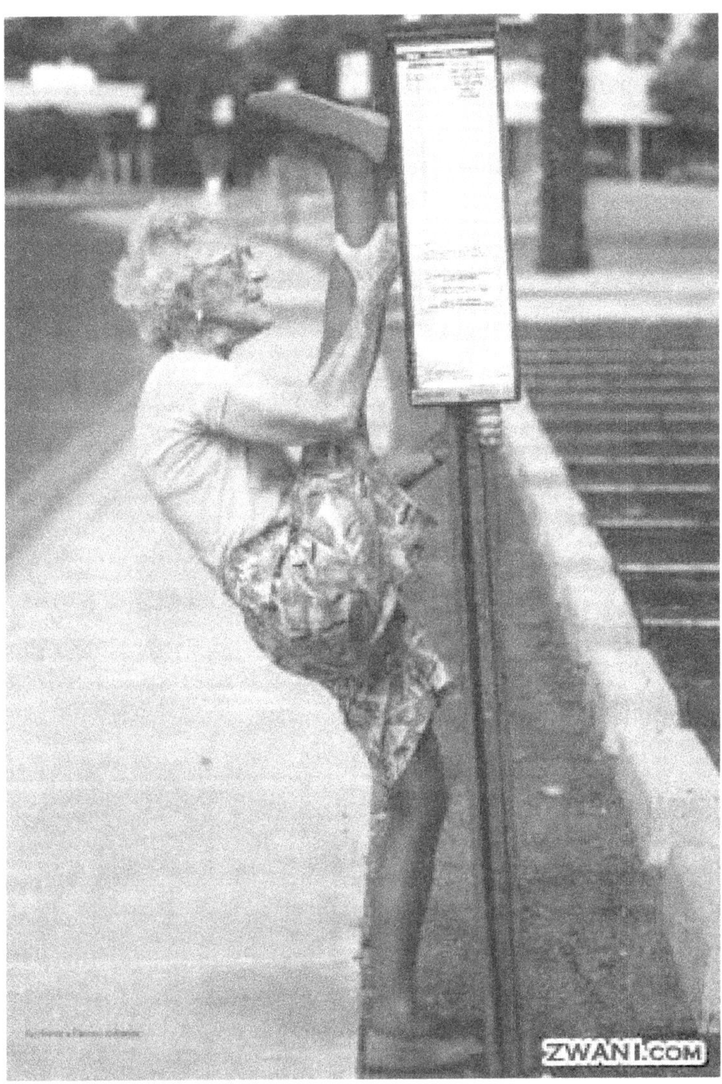

Key Points to Recap:

1. Consistency and regularity are key for reaping the benefits

of Pilates as an elderly beginner.

2. Aim for frequent short sessions rather than sporadic longer ones.

3. Start by dedicating a specific time each day to practice Pilates.

4. Embed Pilates exercises into everyday activities to extend the practice beyond designated workout times.

5. Set achievable goals, track progress, and reward milestones to stay motivated.

6. Engage with a supportive community in person or online for collective encouragement.

7. Consider complementary activities like walking, swimming, or tai chi to supplement your Pilates routine.

8. Every bit of movement counts, and keeping your body engaged will help you get the most out of your Pilates journey.

Addressing Common Questions and Concerns Regarding Practicing Pilates as a Senior

Q1: Is Pilates safe for seniors to practice?**

A1: Yes, Pilates can be a very safe and beneficial form of exercise for seniors. It focuses on controlled movements that can help improve flexibility, core strength, and balance, which are especially important for aging bodies. However, it is essential for seniors to work with a qualified instructor and to consult with healthcare providers before starting any new exercise regimen, especially if there are existing health concerns.

Q2: Can Pilates help with arthritis and joint pain?**

A2: Pilates can be gentle on the joints and may help improve joint mobility and decrease pain caused by arthritis. The low-impact nature of Pilates exercises can help maintain joint health without causing undue stress.

Q3: What if I have a limited range of motion?

A3: Pilates exercises can be modified to accommodate a limited range of motion. Working with an experienced instructor allows for the personalization of the workout to address individual restrictions and to expand flexibility over time safely.

Q4: Am I too old to start Pilates?

A4: There is no age limit for starting Pilates. The practice is adaptable and can be beneficial regardless of when you begin. It's about personal progress, listening to your body, and not competing with others.

Q5: How often should seniors practice Pilates to see benefits?

A5: Consistency is key rather than frequency. Seniors may see benefits from practicing Pilates 2-3 times a week. It's important to allow the body time to rest between sessions.

Addressing Common Challenges and Limitations Faced by Seniors During Pilates Exercises

1. **Balance Difficulties**: Balance can become more challenging with age. Using props like chairs for support can help seniors maintain balance during exercises.

2. **Decreased Core Strength**: Seniors may struggle

with exercises that require strong core muscles. Starting with foundational exercises and progressively increasing difficulty can help build core strength.

3. **Flexibility Issues**: Reduced flexibility is common in seniors. Incorporating gentle stretching and modified positions into the Pilates routine can help increase flexibility.

4. **Comfort on the Mat**: Seniors may find lying on a hard surface uncomfortable. Using extra padding or performing exercises on a chair or raised surface can address this issue.

Tips for Overcoming Obstacles and Continuing to Progress with Pilates Practice

1. **Adapt Exercises**: Work with an instructor to adapt exercises to your needs. Modify movements that cause discomfort or are too challenging.

2. **Listen to Your Body**: How your body feels during and after exercises. If something hurts or feels wrong, stop and seek guidance.

3. **Go at Your Own Pace**: Progress at a pace that feels comfortable. It's not about keeping up with others but about steady, personal improvement.

4. **Set Realistic Goals**: Establish achievable goals based on your abilities. Work towards them gradually and celebrate your progress.

5. **Stay Hydrated and Nourished**: Ensure you drink plenty of water and maintain a healthy diet to support your exercise routine.

6. **Be Patient and Consistent**: Improvements in strength and flexibility will come with time and consistent practice. Patience is essential.

7. **Group Classes vs. Private Sessions**: Consider group classes for the social aspect or private sessions for personalized guidance. Both can be beneficial.

8. **Integrate Mindfulness**: Pilates is not just physical; it's also a mindful practice. Focus on breathing and the mind-body connection to enhance the benefits.

Seniors can practice Pilates safely and effectively by addressing these questions, challenges, and tips. Pilates offers a great way for seniors to stay active, improve overall well-being, and lead a healthy lifestyle as they age.

11

References:

- American Council on Exercise - "The Benefits of Pilates for Older Adults"

Donoyama, N., & Ohkoshi, N. (2012). Effects of Anma therapy (traditional Japanese massage) on body and mind. *Journal of Bodywork and Movement Therapies*, 14(1), 55–64. https://doi.org/10.1016/j.jbmt.2009.06.006

Isacowitz, R. (2014). *Pilates' anatomy*. Human Kinetics.

Kloubec, J. A. (2010). Pilates for improvement of muscle endurance, flexibility, balance, and posture. *Journal of Strength and Conditioning Research*, 24(3), 661–667. https://doi.org/10.1519/JSC.0b013e3181c277a6

Küçükçakır, N., Altan, L., & Korkmaz, N. (2013). Effects of Pilates exercises on functional capacity, flexibility, fatigue, depression and quality of life in female breast cancer patients: A randomized

REFERENCES:

controlled study. *European Journal of Physical and Rehabilitation Medicine*, 49(6), 791–800.

- Mayo Clinic - "Pilates Basics: Benefits of this Core Strengthening Workout"

- National Center for Complementary and Integrative Health - "Pilates: What You Need to Know"

Latey, P. (2001). The Pilates method: History and philosophy. *Journal of Bodywork and Movement Therapies*, 5(4), 275–282. https://doi.org/10.1054/jbmt.2001.0237

Olivarez, S. (2010). Adapting exercise for individuals with non-specific chronic low back pain: A case report. *American Journal of Physical Medicine & Rehabilitation*, 89(4), 331–334. https://doi.org/10.1097/PHM.0b013e3181d3e0ba

Wells, C., Kolt, G. S., & Bialocerkowski, A. (2012). Defining Pilates exercise: A systematic review. *Complementary Therapies in Medicine*, 20(4), 253–262. https://doi.org/10.1016/j.ctim.2011.09.007

12

Conclusion

As the final chapter of "Gentle Pilates for the Golden Years: A Transformative Guide for Seniors" draws to a close, I invite you to pause and reflect on the journey you've embarked upon. Our adventure through these pages was designed not simply to impart knowledge but to sow the seeds of a profound lifestyle transformation—one that germinates within the rich soil of Pilates and blooms into an enriching golden age.

By delving into this guide, you've taken the first steps toward envisioning a future shaped by strength, balance, and a harmonious dialogue between your body and mind. Now, let's amplify that vision with the power of testimony.

Martha's story is a beacon, illuminating the path of transformative success. Her initial skepticism led to a steadfast commitment, resulting in a revival of physical prowess and a newfound community of support. Let her words stir within you a recognition of potential and a rally to action.

We've laid out a road map for progress that extends beyond the confines of this book. Embrace the camaraderie and accountability found in a local Pilates class or online community. Dare to weave the principles of Pilates into the very fabric of your daily life—for it is in these small, incremental steps that the most significant changes are born.

Yet, our discourse wouldn't be complete without a nudge toward the realms of further exploration and engagement:

- Dare to dream of afternoons filled with the energizing flows of a Pilates class and evenings graced by the calm of focused breaths and gentle stretches.
  - Keep your spirit ablaze with stories of others like Martha, who have captured the essence of youth within their golden chapters.
  - Challenge the horizon of your Pilates voyage by considering a teacher who can tailor your experience, perfect your practice, and challenge your limits.

The door to a Pilates lifestyle stands ajar, inviting an embrace of its core tenets across all corners of your day-to-day existence.

The golden years are a crescendo of wisdom and potential in the symphony of life's seasons. The art of Pilates—a subtle yet profound conductor—awaits your lead. So, take the stage gracefully and let the music play, a joyful tune that celebrates the abundance of well-being and the rhythms of a well-lived life.

With each breath and movement, you are curating a future of vitality and independence—a tapestry woven with threads of strength and flexibility, both physical and spiritual.

And so, we part with an invitation, not to an end, but to a bright new beginning. Step forward from the final page of this book, brimming with inspiration, equipped with the tools of transformation, and ready to continue shaping a future where every year shines with the promise of Pilates' perennial spring.

Your journey has just begun. May it be filled with the positivity of healthful strides and the invigoration of endless discovery. Show the world how the golden years are not a time to fade but a stage to outshine. Let the ethos of Pilates guide you to a life of vitality and action.

Embark on this path, dear reader, for the most radiant golden years lie in the potential of each disciplined stretch, each deep breath, and each intentional movement. The page turns, but your odyssey through the golden realm of Pilates flourishes onward.

www.ingramcontent.com/pod-product-compliance
Lightning Source LLC
Chambersburg PA
CBHW061933270726
48660CB00007BA/2708